ANGER MANAGEMENT FOR ADULTS WITH ADHD : *How To Recognize And Manage Explosive Anger*.

Christina R Gibson

Table of Contents

Introduction

Anger management for adults with Attention Deficit Hyperactivity Disorder (ADHD) is a set of strategies that can help individuals better understand and manage their angry emotions. People with ADHD may have more difficulty controlling their anger and may experience more intense feelings of anger than those without the disorder. Anger management techniques can help these individuals learn how to recognize the triggers of their anger, how to use relaxation techniques to calm their bodies and minds, and how to use positive self-talk to reframe their thinking. It may also involve seeking the guidance of a mental health professional to develop a treatment plan and provide additional support. By learning and practicing effective anger management techniques, adults with ADHD can improve their overall well-being and relationships with others.

If left unchecked, anger can lead to conflicts in relationships, problems at work, and even legal issues if not properly managed. While it is natural to feel angry from time to time, it is important for adults with ADHD to learn effective strategies for managing their anger in a healthy way. This is where anger management comes in. Anger management for adults with ADHD is a set of techniques that can help individuals better understand and manage their angry emotions, and improve their overall well-being and relationships with others. In this book, we will discuss the importance of anger management for adults with ADHD, and provide some tips and strategies for effectively managing anger.

Chapter 1: Recognizing The Signs Of Anger In Adults With ADHD

Anger is a normal emotion that everyone experiences from time to time, but for adults with Attention Deficit Hyperactivity Disorder (ADHD), it can be more intense and harder to control. If left unchecked, anger can lead to conflicts in relationships, problems at work, and even legal issues. That's why it's important for adults with ADHD to learn how to recognize the signs of anger in themselves and others, and to develop strategies for managing and reducing it.

The first step in recognizing the signs of anger in adults with ADHD is to understand what anger is and how it manifests. ***Anger is a natural response to a perceived threat or injustice.*** It is a normal and healthy emotion, but it can become a problem when it is intense and difficult to control.

There are several physical, behavioral, and cognitive signs of anger that adults with ADHD should be aware of.
Physical signs of anger may include:

- Increased heart rate- When an individual becomes angry, their heart rate may increase as a result of the body's "fight or flight" response.
- Clenched fists or jaw- Some people may clench their fists or jaw when they are feeling angry.
- Rapid breathing
- Tight muscles- Anger can also cause an individual's muscles to tense up, which may lead to physical discomfort or pain.
- Sweating
- Headaches
- Stomach aches

- Increased blood pressure- Anger can cause an individual's blood pressure to rise, which may lead to headaches or other physical symptoms.

Emotional signs of anger may include:

- Feelings of frustration or irritability: These emotions may be a sign that an individual is feeling angry or upset.
- Short temper: Adults with ADHD may have a shorter temper than those without the disorder, which may cause them to become angry more easily.
- Difficulty controlling emotions: Some adults with ADHD may have trouble controlling their emotions, including anger. They may feel overwhelmed by their emotions and have difficulty calming down.

Behavioral signs of anger may include:

- Yelling or shouting- An individual may become louder or more animated when they are feeling angry. Adults with ADHD may have difficulty controlling their words when they are angry. They may speak loudly or aggressively, or use harsh language.
- Physical aggression, such as hitting or throwing objects- Adults with ADHD may be more prone to this type of behavior due to their impulsivity.
- Arguing or fighting- Anger may cause an individual to become more argumentative or prone to conflict.
- Withdrawing from others or isolating oneself- This can be a sign that they are struggling to manage their anger.
- Engaging in risky or dangerous behavior
- Procrastination or avoidance of tasks

Cognitive signs of anger may include:

- Negative thoughts or beliefs about oneself or others
- Difficulty concentrating
- Impulsive thinking or decision-making
- Difficulty remembering things
- Difficulty processing or expressing emotions

It's important to note that not everyone with ADHD will experience all of these signs of anger, and the intensity and frequency of these signs may vary from person to person. Some individuals may be more prone to physical symptoms of anger, while others may be more emotional or behavioral. It's also worth noting that the intensity of these signs may vary from person to person.

It's also important to remember that anger is a normal and healthy emotion, and it's okay to feel angry from time to time. The key is to learn how to recognize and manage anger in a healthy way. By becoming aware of these emotions, individuals can work to manage their anger before it gets out of control.

One way to recognize the signs of anger in oneself and others is to pay attention to physical cues. If you notice that your heart rate is increasing or your muscles are tense, it may be a sign that you are becoming angry. Similarly, if you notice that someone else is sweating or has a red face, they may be feeling angry.

Another way to recognize the signs of anger is to pay attention to behavioral cues. If you or someone else is yelling or engaging in physical aggression, it may be a sign of anger. Withdrawing from others or engaging in risky behavior can also be signs of anger.

It's also important to pay attention to cognitive cues, such as negative thoughts or impulsive decision-making. These can be indicators that anger is present.

Once you have identified the signs of anger in yourself or others, the next step is to develop strategies for managing and reducing it. There are several effective strategies that adults with ADHD can use to manage their anger and improve their overall well-being.

One strategy is to practice ***relaxation techniques, such as deep breathing, progressive muscle relaxation, and meditation.*** These techniques can help calm the body and mind, and can be especially helpful when you start to feel angry.

Another strategy ***is to use positive self-talk.*** When you're feeling angry, it's easy to get caught up in negative thoughts. Instead, try to reframe your thinking and use positive self-talk to reassure yourself. For example, instead of telling yourself "I can't handle this," try saying "I am capable of managing this situation."

Taking a break can also be helpful when you're feeling overwhelmed by anger. If you're feeling angry, try to remove yourself from the situation for a few minutes.

Chapter 2: Identifying Triggers For Anger In Adults With ADHD

Anger is a normal and healthy emotion that everyone experiences from time to time. However, for adults with Attention Deficit Hyperactivity Disorder (ADHD), managing anger can sometimes be a challenge. This is because ADHD can make it difficult for individuals to regulate their emotions and behaviors. In order to better manage their anger and avoid outbursts or conflicts, it can be helpful for adults with ADHD to identify their triggers for anger.

What are triggers for anger? ***Triggers are anything that causes a person to feel angry or agitated.*** These can be external stimuli, such as certain people or situations, or internal factors, such as feelings of stress or frustration. Triggers for anger can vary widely from person to person, and it's important for individuals to take the time to identify their own unique triggers.

Here are some common triggers for anger in adults with ADHD:

- **Feeling overwhelmed or stressed**: Adults with ADHD may have difficulty managing their time and responsibilities, which can lead to feelings of stress and overwhelm. This can be especially true if they are trying to juggle multiple tasks at once or if they are faced with unexpected challenges or changes in their schedule.

- **Feeling misunderstood or unappreciated**: Adults with ADHD may feel misunderstood or unappreciated by others, which can trigger feelings of anger. This may be because they feel like others don't fully understand their challenges or the way that their brain works, or because they feel like others don't value their contributions.

- **Feelings of failure or inadequacy**: Adults with ADHD may struggle with self-esteem and feelings of inadequacy, which can be triggered by experiences of failure or setbacks. For example, they may feel angry if they make a mistake at work or if they feel like they are falling behind on their goals.

- **Difficulties with time management or organization**: Adults with ADHD may have trouble with time management and organization, which can lead to feelings of frustration and anger. For example, they may feel angry if they are running late for an appointment or if they can't find an important document.

- **Unmet needs or desires**: Adults with ADHD may have unmet needs or desires that can trigger feelings of anger. This may be because they feel like they aren't getting the support or resources they need to succeed, or because they feel like their wants and needs aren't being recognized or respected.

- **Feeling disrespected or mistreated**: Adults with ADHD may feel disrespected or mistreated by others, which can trigger feelings of anger. This may be because they feel like others are being condescending or dismissive, or because they feel like others are taking advantage of them.

- **Physical or mental fatigue**: Adults with ADHD may become more prone to anger when they are physically or mentally exhausted. This is because fatigue can make it harder for them to regulate their emotions and behaviors.

Identifying triggers for anger in adults with ADHD can be a helpful first step in managing this emotion. Once individuals have identified their triggers, they can start to develop strategies for coping with these triggers and preventing anger from escalating. This may include finding ways to reduce stress, setting boundaries with others, and finding healthy outlets for their emotions.

Managing anger is a process that takes time and effort, and it may require individuals to seek support from a mental health professional. With patience and persistence, however, adults with ADHD can learn to better manage their anger and improve their relationships and overall well-being.

It can be helpful for adults with ADHD to identify their triggers for anger.

External triggers for anger are things or situations that occur outside of an individual and can trigger feelings of anger. These triggers can vary widely from person to person, and it's important for individuals to take the time to identify their own unique triggers. Some common external triggers for anger in adults with ADHD include:

- **Certain people or relationships**: Adults with ADHD may become angry when they are around certain people or in certain relationships. For example, they may feel more prone to anger when interacting with a boss or coworker who is demanding or critical.

- **Stressful or overwhelming situations**: Adults with ADHD may become overwhelmed or stressed when faced with challenging or unfamiliar situations. This can trigger feelings of anger and frustration.

- **Disrespect or mistreatment**: Adults with ADHD may feel disrespected or mistreated by others, which can trigger feelings of anger. This may be because they feel like others are being condescending or dismissive, or because they feel like others are taking advantage of them.

- **Changes in routine or expectations**: Adults with ADHD may become agitated or angry when their routine or expectations are disrupted. This may be because they rely on routine and structure to feel grounded and in control.

While external triggers for anger, such as certain people or situations, are often easier to identify and manage, internal triggers for anger can be more challenging to recognize and address. *Internal triggers for anger are thoughts, feelings, or beliefs that arise from within an individual and can trigger feelings of anger. Some common internal triggers for anger in adults with ADHD include:*

- **Negative self-talk**: Adults with ADHD may engage in negative self-talk, such as telling themselves that they are incompetent or unworthy. This negative self-talk can trigger feelings of anger and frustration.

- **Perfectionism**: Adults with ADHD may struggle with perfectionism, which can lead to feelings of anger when they feel like they are falling short of their own expectations.

- **Impulsivity**: Adults with ADHD may have difficulty controlling their impulses, which can lead to impulsive behavior and outbursts of anger.

- **Low self-esteem:** Adults with ADHD may struggle with low self-esteem, which can be triggered by experiences of failure or setbacks. This can lead to feelings of anger and frustration.

- **Difficulty with emotional regulation**: Adults with ADHD may have difficulty regulating their emotions, which can lead to feelings of anger and frustration.

Identifying and addressing internal triggers for anger in adults with ADHD can be a helpful step in managing this emotion. This may involve engaging in self-reflection, seeking support from a mental health professional, or finding healthy ways to cope with and express emotions. With patience and persistence, adults with ADHD can learn to better manage their anger and improve their overall well-being.

Chapter 3: Techniques For Managing And Reducing Anger In Adults With ADHD

Anger is a normal and natural emotion that everyone experiences at some point in their lives. However, for adults with attention deficit hyperactivity disorder (ADHD), managing and reducing anger can be particularly challenging. This is because individuals with ADHD often struggle with impulse control and difficulty regulating their emotions. If left unchecked, anger can lead to negative outcomes such as strained relationships, problems at work, and even physical health problems. Fortunately, there are several techniques that adults with ADHD can use to manage and reduce their anger.

One effective technique is to practice **deep breathing exercises.** When we get angry, our bodies go through a series of physical changes, including an increase in heart rate and blood pressure. Deep breathing helps to regulate these physical responses and can help to calm the body and mind. To practice deep breathing, find a quiet and comfortable place to sit or stand. Take a deep breath in through your nose, filling your lungs with air. Hold the breath for a few seconds, then slowly exhale through your mouth. Repeat this process for several minutes.

To practice deep breathing exercises:

1. Find a quiet and comfortable place to sit or stand. You may want to close your eyes to help you focus on your breathing.

2. Take a deep breath in through your nose, filling your lungs with air. Hold the breath for a few seconds.

3. Exhale slowly through your mouth.

4. Repeat the process for several minutes. You can also try counting to four as you inhale, hold your breath for a count of four, and then exhale for a count of four.

If you find it helpful, you can also try placing one hand on your chest and the other on your stomach. As you inhale, focus on expanding your stomach and feeling your hand rise. As you exhale, feel your hand fall back down. This can help to ensure that you are taking full, deep breaths.

As you practice deep breathing, try to focus your attention on the present moment and the sensation of your breath moving in and out of your body. If you get distracted by thoughts, gently redirect your focus back to your breathing.

Practice deep breathing regularly, perhaps a few times a day. With time and practice, you may find it becomes easier to use deep breathing as a way to calm yourself when you are feeling angry or upset.

Another technique that can be helpful for managing anger is to use **positive self-talk**. When we get angry, it's easy to get caught up in negative thoughts and self-criticism. However, these negative thoughts can actually make our anger worse. Instead, try to reframe your thoughts in a more positive light. For example, instead of telling yourself "I can't believe I messed this up again," try saying "Everyone makes mistakes, and I can learn from this experience." This can help to put things in perspective and reduce the intensity of your anger.

Positive self-talk involves reframing negative thoughts in a more positive light. When we get angry, it's easy to get caught up in negative thoughts and self-criticism, which can make our anger worse. Here are some steps for using positive self-talk to calm anger:

1. Identify the negative thoughts that are contributing to your anger. These may include thoughts such as "I can't believe I messed this up again" or "I'm so stupid."

2. Challenge these negative thoughts by asking yourself if they are really true. Are you really "stupid" because you made a mistake, or is it just a normal part of being human?

3. Reframe the negative thoughts in a more positive way. For example, instead of telling yourself "I can't believe I messed this up again," try saying "Everyone makes mistakes, and I can learn from this experience."

4. Practice using positive self-talk regularly, particularly when you are feeling angry or upset. With time and practice, you may find

that it becomes easier to reframe your thoughts in a more positive light.

It's important to remember that positive self-talk is a skill that can be developed with practice. It may take time and effort to change your thought patterns, but the benefits are worth it. Using positive self-talk can help to reduce the intensity of your anger and improve your overall well-being.

It can also be helpful to find healthy ways to express your anger. Sometimes, bottling up anger can lead to an explosion of emotions later on. Instead, try to find healthy ways to let off steam. This could include going for a run, writing in a journal, or talking to a trusted friend or family member. It's important to find activities that work for you and that you find enjoyable.

Another strategy that can be particularly effective for managing anger in adults with ADHD is to use **a "cool-down" period**.

This involves taking a break from the situation that is causing you to feel angry and giving yourself time to calm down. During this time, you can try some of the techniques mentioned above, such as deep breathing or positive self-talk. It's important to have a specific plan in place for how you will use your cool-down period, whether it's going for a walk or taking a few minutes to meditate.

The "cool-down" period is a technique that involves taking a break from the situation that is causing you to feel angry and giving yourself time to calm down. Here are some steps for using the cool-down period in anger management:

1. Identify the triggers that lead to your anger. These may include specific people, situations, or events that cause you to feel angry.

2. When you start to feel angry, take a step back from the situation and remove yourself from the trigger if possible. This could involve physically leaving the room or taking a break from the activity.

3. During your cool-down period, try some relaxation techniques such as deep breathing or positive self-talk to help calm your body and mind.

Have a specific plan in place for how you will use your cool-down period. This could include going for a walk, taking a few minutes to meditate, or engaging in a hobby or activity that you enjoy.

Once you have had a chance to cool down, revisit the situation that was causing your anger. Try to approach it with a clear head and a more rational perspective.

It's important to remember that the cool-down period is not a way to avoid dealing with your anger. Instead, it is a way to give yourself time to calm down and better regulate your emotions so that you can approach the situation in a more productive and healthy way. With practice, the cool-down period can be a valuable tool for managing and reducing anger.

Finally, it can be helpful to seek professional help if your anger is causing significant problems in your life. A mental health professional, such as a therapist or counselor, can help you to better understand the root causes of your anger and develop strategies for managing it. They can also help you to identify any underlying issues, such as depression or anxiety, that may be contributing to your anger.

In conclusion, managing and reducing anger can be a challenging task for adults with ADHD. However, with practice and the use of techniques such as deep breathing, positive self-talk, and a cool-down period, it is possible to improve impulse control and better regulate emotions. If needed, seeking the help of a mental health professional can also be an effective way to manage and reduce anger.

Chapter 4: The Role Of positive self-talk In Anger Management For Adults With ADHD

Positive self-talk is a technique that involves reframing negative thoughts in a more positive light. It can be a particularly useful tool for adults with attention deficit hyperactivity disorder (ADHD) to use in anger management. This is because individuals with ADHD often struggle with impulse control and difficulty regulating their emotions. Negative self-talk can make it harder to manage anger and can lead to negative outcomes such as strained relationships, problems at work, and even physical health problems. On the other hand, positive self-talk can help to reduce the intensity of anger and improve overall well-being.

When we get angry, it's easy to get caught up in negative thoughts and self-criticism. For example, someone with ADHD may think "I can't believe I messed this up again," which can make their anger worse. However, by reframing this thought in a more positive way, such as "Everyone makes mistakes, and I can learn from this experience," it can help to put things in perspective and reduce the intensity of the anger.

Using positive self-talk can be particularly helpful for adults with ADHD because it helps to improve impulse control and regulate emotions. When we are able to change our thought patterns, it can have a positive effect on our behavior and our overall well-being.

One way to practice positive self-talk is to set aside a few minutes each day to **write down any negative thoughts that come to mind and reframe them** in a more positive way. For example, instead of telling yourself "I'm so clumsy," try saying "I'm not perfect, but that's okay. Everyone makes mistakes." Over time, this practice can help to change negative thought patterns and improve impulse control and emotional regulation.

Another way to use positive self-talk in anger management is to **have a few positive phrases that you can repeat to yourself when you start to feel angry**. For example, you could try saying "I am in control of my emotions" or "I can handle this situation." These phrases can help to refocus your thoughts and remind you that you have the power to manage your anger.

In conclusion, positive self-talk can be a powerful tool for managing and reducing anger in adults with ADHD. By reframing negative thoughts in a more positive light and practicing positive self-talk regularly, individuals with ADHD can improve impulse control and better regulate their emotions. This can lead to improved relationships, better performance at work, and overall improved well-being.

Effective communication is an important skill for everyone, but it can be particularly challenging for adults with attention deficit hyperactivity disorder (ADHD). This is because individuals with ADHD often struggle with impulse control and difficulty regulating their emotions. In situations that may trigger anger, it can be easy to react impulsively and say or do things that we later regret. However, with practice, it is possible to communicate effectively and assertively, even in situations that may trigger anger.

Here are some tips for communicating effectively and assertively in situations that may trigger anger in adults with ADHD:

1. Take a deep breath and try to calm yourself before speaking. This can help to regulate your emotions and give you a chance to think before you react.

2. Use "I" statements to express your feelings and needs. For example, instead of saying "You're wrong," try saying "I feel frustrated when I feel like my perspective is not being considered." This helps to make it clear that you are expressing your own feelings, rather than attacking the other person.

3. Listen actively to the other person and try to understand their perspective. This involves paying attention to what the other person is saying and asking clarifying questions. This can help to reduce the risk of misunderstandings and conflict.

4. Be open to compromise. While it's important to assert your own needs and boundaries, it's also important to be willing

to find solutions that work for everyone. This may involve finding a middle ground or finding ways to meet each other's needs.

5. Use nonverbal communication effectively. Your body language, facial expressions, and tone of voice can all play a role in how your message is received. Make sure that your nonverbal communication is consistent with what you are trying to say.

6. Practice assertiveness in low-stakes situations. It can be helpful to practice assertiveness in low-stakes situations, such as asking a store clerk for help or requesting a change at a restaurant, before moving on to more challenging situations.
Set boundaries: It's important to set boundaries in relationships to protect your time and energy. This can include saying no to unreasonable requests and taking breaks when you need them.

7. Seek help if needed: If you're struggling to manage your anger in relationships, consider seeking the help of a mental health professional. They can provide support and guidance to help you improve your anger management skills.

8. Apologize when appropriate: If you've lost your temper in a relationship, it's important to apologize and make amends if necessary. This can help repair the relationship and maintain a sense of trust and respect

By following these tips, adults with ADHD can learn to communicate effectively and assertively, even in situations that may trigger anger. With practice, you can develop the skills you need to effectively express your needs and boundaries, and to better manage your emotions. This can lead to improved relationships and better overall well-being

Chapter 5: The Benefits Of Anger Management For Adults With ADHD

There are several reasons why anger management is important for adults with Attention Deficit Hyperactivity Disorder (ADHD). Some of the main reasons include:

1. **Improved relationships:** Uncontrolled anger can lead to conflicts in personal and professional relationships. By learning how to manage anger, adults with ADHD can improve their relationships with friends, family, and colleagues.

Here are some ways that anger management can improve relationships in people with Attention Deficit Hyperactivity Disorder (ADHD):

Improved communication: By learning how to manage anger, individuals with ADHD may be better able to communicate their needs and concerns without becoming angry or aggressive. This can lead to more open and honest communication in relationships.

Enhanced empathy: Anger management techniques can help individuals with ADHD develop a better understanding of other people's emotions and perspectives. This can lead to more empathy and a greater ability to respond to others in a more compassionate and understanding way.

Stronger bonds: When individuals with ADHD are able to manage their anger, they may be more likely to form and maintain strong, positive relationships. This is because people are more likely to want to be around others who are able to regulate their emotions and handle conflicts in a healthy way.

Reduced conflicts: Uncontrolled anger can lead to conflicts and misunderstandings in relationships. By learning how to manage anger, individuals with ADHD may be able to reduce the number and severity of conflicts in their relationships.

Improved intimacy: Effective anger management can lead to a greater sense of emotional intimacy and connection in relationships. When individuals with ADHD are able to manage their anger and communicate more effectively, it can create a stronger sense of trust and intimacy in the relationship.

Overall, anger management can have a positive impact on relationships for individuals with ADHD by improving communication, enhancing empathy, strengthening bonds, reducing conflicts, and improving intimacy.

2. Increased productivity: Anger can be a distraction and can interfere with productivity at work or school. By managing anger, adults with ADHD may be able to focus better and be more productive.

Here are some ways that anger management can help to increase productivity in adults with Attention Deficit Hyperactivity Disorder (ADHD):

Improved focus: Anger can be a distraction and can interfere with focus and productivity. By learning how to manage anger, individuals with ADHD may be able to better focus on their tasks and be more productive.

Enhanced problem-solving skills: Anger management techniques can help individuals with ADHD develop better problem-solving skills and find more effective ways of coping with challenges and stressors. This can lead to increased productivity and better decision-making.

Greater efficiency: When individuals with ADHD are able to manage their anger, they may be more efficient in their work or school tasks. This is because anger can often lead to procrastination and a lack of motivation.

Improved time management: Effective anger management can also help individuals with ADHD improve their time management skills. By learning how to regulate their emotions, they may be better able to prioritize tasks and use their time more efficiently.

Enhanced teamwork: Uncontrolled anger can lead to conflicts in the workplace and can interfere with teamwork. By learning how to manage anger, individuals with ADHD may be able to work more effectively in a team setting and contribute to a positive work environment.

Overall, anger management can help to increase productivity in adults with ADHD by improving focus, enhancing problem-solving skills, increasing efficiency, improving time management, and promoting teamwork.

3. Decreased stress: Chronic anger can contribute to stress and other negative emotions. By managing anger, adults with ADHD may be able to reduce their overall stress levels and improve their mental and emotional well-being.

Anger management can help to decrease stress in adults with Attention Deficit Hyperactivity Disorder (ADHD) in several ways:

Improved coping skills: Anger management techniques can help individuals with ADHD develop better coping skills for handling stressors and challenges. This can lead to a decrease in stress levels.

Enhanced emotional regulation: Effective anger management can also help individuals with ADHD better regulate their emotions, including their anger. This can lead to a reduction in stress and negative emotions.

Increased relaxation: Relaxation techniques, such as deep breathing, progressive muscle relaxation, and meditation, are often used as part of anger management. These techniques can help individuals with ADHD relax and reduce their stress levels.

Improved relationships: Chronic anger can lead to conflicts in relationships, which can be a source of stress. By learning how to manage anger, individuals with ADHD may be able to improve their relationships and decrease the amount of stress they experience.

Enhanced overall well-being: Effective anger management can lead to a number of positive benefits, including improved relationships, increased productivity, and decreased stress. All of these things can contribute to a better overall quality of life and a decrease in stress.

4. Legal problems: Uncontrolled anger can sometimes lead to legal issues, such as assault or property damage. By learning how to manage anger, adults with ADHD can avoid legal problems and potential consequences.

Uncontrolled anger can sometimes lead to legal issues, such as assault or property damage. Here are some ways that anger management can help prevent legal issues in adults with Attention Deficit Hyperactivity Disorder (ADHD):

Improved impulse control: Individuals with ADHD may have more difficulty controlling their impulses, including their anger. Anger management techniques can help individuals with ADHD develop better impulse control and make more thoughtful decisions.

Enhanced communication skills: Effective anger management can also help individuals with ADHD improve their communication skills. This can help them express their needs and concerns in a more appropriate and effective way, rather than resorting to anger or aggression.

Increased awareness of triggers: By learning about their triggers for anger, individuals with ADHD can become more aware of situations that may lead to outbursts of anger. This can help them plan ahead and find ways to cope with these triggers, which can prevent legal issues.

Greater self-regulation: Effective anger management can also help individuals with ADHD develop better self-regulation skills. This can involve learning how to recognize when they are becoming angry and finding ways to calm down before their anger becomes out of control.

By learning and practicing anger management techniques, adults with ADHD can improve their impulse control, communication skills, awareness of triggers, and self-regulation, which can all help prevent legal issues.

5. Improved overall well-being: Effective anger management can lead to a number of positive benefits, including improved relationships, increased productivity, decreased stress, and avoidance of legal problems. All of these things can contribute to a better overall quality of life.

Effective anger management can lead to a number of positive benefits that can contribute to an improvement in overall well-being for adults with Attention Deficit Hyperactivity Disorder (ADHD). Some examples of how anger management can help improve overall well-being include:

Improved mental and emotional health: Chronic anger can contribute to mental and emotional health issues, such as anxiety and depression. By learning how to manage anger, individuals with ADHD may be able to reduce their risk of developing these problems and improve their overall mental and emotional health.

Enhanced physical health: Anger has been linked to a number of physical health problems, such as high blood pressure and heart disease. By learning how to manage anger, individuals with ADHD may be able to reduce their risk of these health problems and improve their overall physical health.

Improved sleep: Anger can interfere with sleep, which can have a negative impact on overall well-being. By learning how to manage anger, individuals with ADHD may be able to sleep better and wake up feeling more rested and refreshed.

Improved relationships: Uncontrolled anger can lead to conflicts in personal and professional relationships. By learning how to manage anger, individuals with ADHD may be able to improve their relationships with friends, family, and colleagues, which can contribute to a sense of overall well-being.

Increased productivity: Effective anger management can also lead to increased productivity at work or school, which can contribute to a sense of accomplishment and overall well-being.

Overall, anger management can help improve overall well-being for adults with ADHD by improving mental and emotional health, enhancing physical health, improving sleep, improving relationships, and increasing productivity.

In summary, anger management is important for adults with ADHD because it can help improve relationships, increase productivity, decrease stress, and avoid legal problems, leading to an overall improvement in well-being.

Chapter 6: The Role Of Medication In Managing Anger In Adults with ADHD

Medication can play an important role in managing anger in adults with attention deficit hyperactivity disorder (ADHD). Here are some ways that medication can help:

1. *Improving impulse control*: ADHD medication can help to improve impulse control, which can reduce the risk of acting on anger impulsively. Medication can help to improve impulse control in individuals with attention deficit hyperactivity disorder (ADHD) by balancing the levels of certain neurotransmitters in the brain. Neurotransmitters are chemical messengers that help to transmit signals between nerve cells. In individuals with ADHD, there may be an imbalance of neurotransmitters, which can lead to problems with impulse control.

ADHD medication works by increasing the levels of certain neurotransmitters, such as dopamine and norepinephrine, which can help to improve focus, concentration, and impulse control. By balancing the levels of these neurotransmitters, medication can help to improve impulse control and reduce the risk of acting on impulses, such as anger, impulsively.

Here are some examples of medications that can help to improve impulse control:

Stimulants:

Stimulant medications, such as amphetamines (e.g. Adderall) and methylphenidates (e.g. Ritalin), are the most commonly used medications for treating ADHD. They work by increasing the levels of neurotransmitters such as dopamine and norepinephrine, which can help to improve focus, concentration, and impulse control.

Non-stimulants: Non-stimulant medications, such as atomoxetine (e.g. Strattera), work by increasing the levels of norepinephrine in the brain, which can help to improve focus, concentration, and impulse control.

Antidepressants: Antidepressant medications, such as tricyclic antidepressants (e.g. Imipramine) and selective serotonin reuptake inhibitors (e.g. Fluoxetine), can also be used to treat ADHD in some cases. They work by increasing the levels of neurotransmitters such as serotonin and norepinephrine, which can help to improve focus, concentration, and impulse control.

2. *Some ADHD medications can help to regulate emotions, which can make it easier to manage anger:* Medication can help regulate the emotions of an adult with ADHD by reducing impulsive behavior and increasing the

ability to focus and control their thoughts and actions. There are several types of medication that are commonly used to treat ADHD in adults, including stimulants like amphetamine and methylphenidate, and non-stimulant medications like atomoxetine and guanfacine. These medications work by affecting the levels of certain chemicals in the brain, such as dopamine and norepinephrine, which play a role in mood and attention.

There are several types of medication that can be used to regulate emotions in adults. These include:

- ***Selective serotonin reuptake inhibitors (SSRIs):*** These are a type of antidepressant that can help improve mood and reduce anxiety. Examples include fluoxetine (Prozac), sertraline (Zoloft), and paroxetine (Paxil).

- *Serotonin-norepinephrine reuptake inhibitors (SNRIs):* These are another type of antidepressant that can also help with mood and anxiety. Examples include venlafaxine (Effexor) and duloxetine (Cymbalta).

- *Atypical Antipsychotics*: These medications can be used to treat a variety of conditions, including depression, anxiety, and bipolar disorder. They can also help with agitation and irritability. Examples include aripiprazole (Abilify), olanzapine (Zyprexa), and risperidone (Risperdal).

- *Mood stabilizers:* These medications can be used to treat conditions such as bipolar disorder, which involves extreme shifts in mood. Examples include lithium, valproic acid (Depakote), and carbamazepine (Tegretol).

It's important to note that these medications can have side effects, and it's important to work with a healthcare provider to find the right medication and dosage for your needs.

3. ***Improving focus and concentration***: ADHD medication can help to improve focus and concentration, which can make it easier to stay on task and avoid situations that may trigger anger.
Medication can help improve focus and concentration in adults with ADHD by affecting the levels of certain chemicals in the brain, such as dopamine and norepinephrine. These chemicals play a role in attention and focus, and medications for ADHD work by increasing the availability of these chemicals in the brain.

There are several types of medication that are commonly used to treat ADHD in adults.

These medications can help reduce impulsive behavior and improve the ability to focus and concentrate on tasks.

It's important to note that medication is only one aspect of treatment for ADHD and is often most effective when used in combination with other treatments, such as therapy and lifestyle changes.
There are several types of medication that can be used to improve focus and concentration in adults with ADHD. These include:

Stimulants: These are the most commonly used medications for ADHD. They work by increasing the availability of dopamine and norepinephrine in the brain, which can help improve focus and concentration. Examples of stimulants include amphetamine (Adderall), methylphenidate (Ritalin), and dextroamphetamine (Dexedrine).

Non-stimulants: These medications can also be used to treat ADHD and can be a good option for people who cannot tolerate stimulants or do not respond well to them. Examples of non-stimulants include atomoxetine (Strattera) and guanfacine (Intuniv).

The medications that can be used to improve focus and concentration in adults with ADHD are generally the same regardless of whether or not the person is angry.

It's important to note that these medications can have side effects, and it's important to work with a healthcare provider to find the right medication and dosage for your needs. In addition, it's important to address the underlying causes of anger, such as stress, frustration, or other emotions, as part of a comprehensive treatment plan. This may involve therapy, lifestyle changes, or other interventions in addition to medication. It's also important to work closely with a healthcare provider to find the right medication and dosage, as well as to monitor for any side effects.

4. ***Reducing hyperactivity:*** Some ADHD medications can help to reduce hyperactivity, which can make it easier to manage anger and other emotions.

Chapter 7: Strategies For Maintaining Progress in Anger Management Over Time In Adults with ADHD

Anger is a common issue for adults with ADHD, and managing it can be a lifelong challenge. While medication and therapy can be helpful in the short term, it's important to have strategies in place to maintain progress over the long term. Here are some tips for maintaining progress in anger management over time in adults with ADHD:

1. Practice relaxation techniques: Relaxation is the state of feeling calm and at ease, and it can be helpful in reducing stress, anxiety, and anger. Learning relaxation techniques such as deep breathing, meditation, or progressive muscle relaxation can help you manage your anger in the moment. Practice these techniques regularly to make them second nature when you need them.

2. **Identify triggers**: Take some time to think about what triggers your anger and try to avoid those situations or find healthy ways to cope with them. There are many different things that can trigger anger in people with ADHD. Some common triggers include:

Stress: Stressful situations or events can easily trigger anger in people with ADHD.

Frustration: Difficulty completing tasks or understanding instructions can lead to frustration, which can in turn lead to anger.

Disorganization: Struggling to keep track of things and maintain organization can be a major source of frustration and anger for people with ADHD.

Confusion: Not understanding something or feeling overwhelmed can lead to confusion and frustration, which can trigger anger.

Impulsivity: Difficulty controlling impulsive behavior can lead to situations that trigger anger.

Interpersonal conflicts: Difficulties in relationships, whether at home or at work, can be a common trigger for anger in people with ADHD.

By identifying your own triggers and working with a therapist or coach, you can learn to manage your anger and find healthy ways to cope with these triggers

3. **Communicate effectively:** Use "I" statements to express your feelings and needs, and try to listen actively to others to improve your communication and reduce

misunderstandings.   Effective communication is an important skill that can help improve relationships and reduce conflict. Here are some tips for communicating effectively:

Use "I" statements: When expressing your feelings or needs, try to use "I" statements to describe how you feel and what you need. This helps to avoid blame and can make it easier for the other person to understand your perspective.

Listen actively: Pay attention to what the other person is saying, and try to understand their perspective. Use nonverbal cues like nodding your head and making eye contact to show that you're listening.

Avoid interrupting: Allow the other person to finish speaking before you respond. This shows respect and helps to avoid misunderstandings.

Stay calm: It's natural to get emotional when discussing sensitive topics, but try to stay as calm as possible. Take deep breaths and try to keep your voice at a normal volume.

Use "we" statements: When working on a problem or trying to find a solution, try to use "we" statements to show that you're working together. This helps to build collaboration and trust.

By following these tips, you can improve your communication skills and build stronger, more positive relationships

4. Find healthy ways to cope with stress: Stress is a common trigger for anger, so finding healthy ways to cope with stress, such as exercise, hobbies, or talking to a friend, can be helpful in managing anger. There are many healthy ways to cope with stress, and what works for one person may not work for another. Here are a few ideas to try:

Exercise: Physical activity can help reduce stress and improve mood. It can be as simple as taking a walk, going for a run, or participating in a favorite sport.

Practice relaxation techniques: Techniques such as deep breathing, meditation, or progressive muscle relaxation can help reduce stress and promote feelings of calm.

Get enough sleep: Lack of sleep can contribute to stress, so it's important to get enough rest. Try to establish a regular sleep schedule and create a relaxing bedtime routine.

Eat a healthy diet: A balanced diet that includes plenty of fruits, vegetables, and whole grains can help reduce stress and improve overall health.

Engage in activities you enjoy: Doing things you enjoy, such as hobbies or creative pursuits, can help reduce stress and improve your mood.

Connect with others: Social support is important for managing stress. Consider reaching out to friends, family, or a therapist for support and guidance.

Seek professional help: If stress is causing significant problems in your life, it may be helpful to seek the help of a mental health professional. A therapist can provide support and guidance to help you manage stress and improve your overall well-being.

5. Seek support: Don't be afraid to reach out to friends, family, or a therapist for support and guidance. They can provide a listening ear and help you brainstorm solutions to challenges.

Friends and family: Talk to your loved ones about your struggles with ADHD and how they can support you. They may be able to offer practical assistance, such as help with organization or scheduling, or just be a listening ear when you need to vent.

Support groups: There are many support groups for adults with ADHD, both in-person and online. These groups can provide a sense of community and a place to share experiences and strategies for managing ADHD.

Therapists or coaches: A therapist or coach who specializes in ADHD can provide support and guidance to help you manage your symptoms and improve your overall well-being.

Doctors: Talk to your primary care doctor or a specialist about your concerns and ask for recommendations for treatment and support.

Employee assistance programs: Many companies offer employee assistance programs that provide resources and support for employees dealing with personal or mental health issues. If you're struggling with ADHD at work, this can be a good place to start.

By seeking support from these sources, you can get the help you need to manage your ADHD and improve your overall well-being

6. Practice self-care: Take care of your physical and emotional health by getting enough sleep, eating a healthy diet, and engaging in activities that bring you joy and relaxation. Self-care is the practice of taking care of your own physical, mental, and emotional health. It's an important aspect of overall well-being, and it's especially important for people with ADHD, who may face additional challenges in managing their health and well-being. Here are some tips for practicing self-care:

Get enough sleep: Sleep is important for physical and mental health, and it can be especially challenging for people with ADHD to get enough rest. Establish a regular sleep schedule and create a relaxing bedtime routine to help improve your sleep.

Eat a healthy diet: A balanced diet that includes plenty of fruits, vegetables, and whole grains can help improve your physical and mental health. Avoid sugary or processed foods, which can contribute to mood and energy fluctuations.

Exercise regularly: Physical activity can help reduce stress and improve mood. Aim for at least 30 minutes of moderate-intensity activity, such as a brisk walk or bike ride, most days of the week.

Engage in activities you enjoy: Doing things you enjoy, such as hobbies or creative pursuits, can help reduce stress and improve your mood.

Connect with others: Social support is important for overall well-being. Make time to spend with friends and family, and consider joining a support group or connecting with others who have similar interests.

Practice relaxation techniques: Techniques such as deep breathing, meditation, or progressive muscle relaxation can help reduce stress and promote feelings of calm.

By incorporating these self-care practices into your daily routine, you can improve your overall well-being and better manage the challenges of ADHD.

Incorporating these strategies into your daily routine, you can maintain progress in anger management over time and live a happier, healthier life.

Chapter 8: Seeking Professional Help for Anger Management In Adults With ADHD

If you're struggling to manage your anger as an adult with ADHD, it may be helpful to seek the help of a mental health professional. Anger management is an important aspect of treatment for ADHD, and a therapist or coach can provide support and guidance to help you learn healthy ways to cope with your anger.

There are several different approaches that a mental health professional might use to help you manage your anger. These may include:

Cognitive-behavioral therapy: This type of therapy helps you identify negative thought patterns that contribute to your anger and teaches you new ways of thinking and behaving. Cognitive-behavioral therapy (CBT) is a type of psychotherapy that focuses on helping you identify and change negative thought patterns and behaviors that contribute to your problems. It's a popular and effective treatment for a wide range of issues, including anger management.

During CBT, you'll work with a therapist to identify your negative thought patterns and the behaviors that result from them. You'll then learn new ways of thinking and behaving that can help you better manage your emotions and behavior.

CBT is a short-term treatment that typically lasts for several months. It can be done individually or in a group setting. It's a structured approach that involves setting specific goals and working towards them through a series of sessions.

CBT can be an effective treatment for anger management because it helps you identify and change the negative thought patterns that contribute to your anger. It also teaches you new coping skills and strategies for managing your anger in healthy ways.

If you're struggling to manage your anger and are interested in trying CBT, it's important to find a qualified therapist who is trained in this approach. Together, you can develop a treatment plan that meets your specific needs and helps you learn healthy ways to cope with your anger.

There are many different types of cognitive-behavioral therapy (CBT), and the approach that is best for you will depend on your needs and preferences. Here are a few examples of different types of CBT:

Cognitive-behavioral therapy for depression: This type of CBT focuses on helping you identify and change negative thought patterns and behaviors that contribute to depression.

Cognitive-behavioral therapy for anxiety: This type of CBT helps you identify and change negative thought patterns and behaviors that contribute to anxiety.

Cognitive-behavioral therapy for insomnia: This type of CBT helps you identify and change negative thought patterns and behaviors that contribute to insomnia.

Cognitive-behavioral therapy for anger management: This type of CBT helps you identify and change negative thought patterns and behaviors that contribute to anger.

Dialectical behavior therapy: This type of therapy focuses on helping you develop skills to manage strong emotions, such as anger. Dialectical behavior therapy (DBT) is a type of psychotherapy that was developed to help people who struggle with strong emotions, such as anger. It's a form of cognitive-behavioral therapy that focuses on helping you develop skills to manage your emotions and improve your relationships.

DBT was originally developed to treat borderline personality disorder, but it has since been found to be effective for a wide range of issues, including anger management.

During DBT, you'll work with a therapist to learn new skills for managing your emotions and improving your relationships. These skills can include mindfulness, emotion regulation, and distress tolerance.

DBT is a structured treatment that involves weekly individual therapy sessions and weekly skills training groups. It's a short-term treatment that typically lasts for several months.

One of the key components of DBT is mindfulness, which involves being present in the moment and accepting your thoughts and feelings without judgment. This can be helpful in managing anger because it helps you become more aware of your emotions and how to respond to them in a healthy way.

If you're struggling to manage your anger and are interested in trying DBT, it's important to find a qualified therapist who is trained in this approach. Together, you can develop a treatment plan that meets your specific needs and helps you learn healthy ways to cope with your anger.

There are several different types of dialectical behavior therapy (DBT), and the approach that is best for you will depend on your needs and preferences. Here are a few examples of different types of DBT:

Individual DBT: This type of DBT involves working one-on-one with a therapist to learn skills for managing emotions and improving relationships.

Group DBT: This type of DBT involves attending skills training groups with a group of people who are dealing with similar issues. It can provide a sense of community and support, and it can be helpful in managing anger because it allows you to see that you're not alone in your struggles.

Phone coaching: This type of DBT involves working with a therapist over the phone to practice skills and get support between sessions.

Online DBT: This type of DBT involves participating in skills training and therapy sessions online. It can be a convenient option for people who have difficulty accessing in-person treatment.

Mindfulness-based therapy: This type of therapy teaches you to be more aware of your thoughts and feelings in the present moment and to respond to them in a more mindful and effective way. Mindfulness-based therapy is a type of psychotherapy that involves training in mindfulness, which is the practice of being present in the moment and accepting your thoughts and feelings without judgment. It's a form of cognitive-behavioral therapy that can be helpful in managing anger because it helps you become more aware of your emotions and how to respond to them in a healthy way.

During mindfulness-based therapy, you'll work with a therapist to learn mindfulness techniques, such as deep breathing and meditation, that can help you manage your emotions and reduce stress. You'll also learn to recognize and challenge negative thought patterns that contribute to your anger.

Mindfulness-based therapy is typically a short-term treatment that lasts for several months. It can be done individually or in a group setting.

One of the benefits of mindfulness-based therapy is that it can be practiced outside of therapy sessions, which can help you maintain the skills you learn over time.

If you're struggling to manage your anger and are interested in trying mindfulness-based therapy, it's important to find a qualified therapist who is trained in this approach. Together, you can develop a treatment plan that meets your specific needs and helps you learn healthy ways to cope with your anger.

There are many different types of mindfulness-based therapy, and the approach that is best for you will depend on your needs and preferences. Here are a few examples of different types of mindfulness-based therapy:

Mindfulness-based cognitive therapy: This type of therapy combines mindfulness techniques with cognitive-behavioral therapy to help you identify and change negative thought patterns that contribute to your problems.

Mindfulness-based stress reduction: This type of therapy involves a structured program of mindfulness practices, such as meditation and yoga, to help reduce stress and improve overall well-being.

Acceptance and commitment therapy: This type of therapy combines mindfulness with behavioral and cognitive techniques to help you accept your thoughts and feelings and take action to make positive changes in your life.

Dialectical behavior therapy: This type of therapy combines mindfulness with cognitive-behavioral therapy to help you develop skills to manage your emotions and improve your relationships.

Supportive therapy: A therapist can provide a safe and supportive space to discuss your anger and other emotions, and help you develop strategies to cope with them. Supportive therapy is a type of psychotherapy that focuses on providing a safe and supportive environment for you to discuss your emotions and challenges. It's a non-judgmental approach that can be helpful in managing anger because it allows you to express your feelings and work through them in a supportive and accepting environment.

During supportive therapy, you'll work with a therapist to identify your feelings and thoughts about your anger and to develop strategies for managing it in healthy ways. Your therapist will listen and offer guidance and support, but they won't try to direct you or tell you what to do.

Supportive therapy can be a short-term or long-term treatment, depending on your needs. It can be done individually or in a group setting.

One of the benefits of supportive therapy is that it can provide a sense of community and connection, which can be especially helpful for people who are struggling with anger.

If you're struggling to manage your anger and are interested in trying supportive therapy, it's important to find a qualified therapist who is trained in this approach. Together, you can develop a treatment plan that meets your specific needs and helps you learn healthy ways to cope with your anger.

Seeking professional help can be a helpful step in managing your anger and improving your overall well-being. A mental health professional can work with you to develop a treatment plan that meets your specific needs and helps you learn healthy ways to cope with your anger.

There are many different types of supportive therapy, and the approach that is best for you will depend on your needs and preferences. Here are a few examples of different types of supportive therapy:

Psychodynamic therapy: This type of supportive therapy focuses on helping you understand the unconscious thoughts and feelings that contribute to your emotions and behaviors.

Person-centered therapy: This type of supportive therapy emphasizes your own thoughts and feelings, and the therapist provides a non-judgmental and accepting environment for you to explore them.

Group therapy: This type of supportive therapy involves meeting with a group of people who are dealing with similar issues. It can provide a sense of community and support, and it can be helpful in managing anger because it allows you to see that you're not alone in your struggles.

Family therapy: This type of supportive therapy involves working with your family to address and resolve conflicts or issues that may be contributing to your anger.

Couples therapy: This type of supportive therapy involves working with your partner to improve communication and resolve conflicts that may be contributing to your anger.

By working with a qualified therapist, you can determine the type of supportive therapy that is best suited to your needs and goals.